KETO LOW-CARB DIET

A Ketogenic Diet to Lose Weight and Fight Metabolic Disease

Lory Ason

Copyright © 2021 Lory Ason

CONTENTS

THE COMPLETE GUIDE FOR STARTING A
Keto or Low Carb Diet

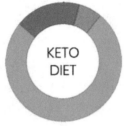

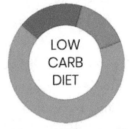

KETO DIET

LOW CARB DIET

| 5-10% carbs | 20-25% protein | 60-75% fat | 15-30% carbs | 15-30% protein | 40-70% fat |

WHAT TO EAT:

- Healthy Fats
- Eggs
- Meat
- Poultry
- Seafood

- Full-fat Dairy
- Nuts & Seeds
- Leafy Greens
- Low Carb Veggies
- Berries

BREAD PASTA SUGAR MILK CORN BEANS RICE

1. PORK LOIN STEAKS IN CREAMY PEPPER SAUCE

Preparation Time: 15 minutes

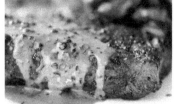

Cooking Time: 10 minutes

Servings: 2

Ingredients:

1 teaspoon lard, at room temperature

2 pork loin steaks

1/2 cup beef bone broth

2 bell peppers, deseeded and chopped

1 shallot, chopped

1 garlic clove, minced

Sea salt, to season

1/2 teaspoon cayenne pepper

1/4 teaspoon paprika

1 teaspoon Italian seasoning mix

1/4 cup Greek-style yogurt

Kitchen Equipment:

cast-iron skillet

Directions:

Melt the lard in a cast-iron skillet over moderate heat. Once hot, cook the pork loin steaks until slightly browned or approximately 5 minutes per side; reserve.

Add a splash of the beef bone broth to deglaze the pan. Now, cook the bell peppers, shallot, and garlic until tender and aromatic—season with salt, cayenne pepper, paprika, and Italian seasoning mix.

After that, decrease the temperature to medium-low, add the Greek yogurt to the skillet and let it simmer for 2 minutes more or until heated through. Serve immediately.

Nutrition: **Calories** 447 - **Fat**19.2g - **Protein:** 62.2g

2. PORK MEDALLIONS WITH CABBAGE

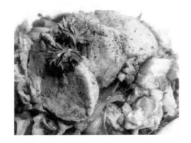

Preparation Time: 20 minutes

Cooking Time: 15 minutes

Servings: 2

Ingredients:

Ingredients

1ounce bacon, diced

2 pork medallions

2 garlic cloves, sliced

1 red onion, chopped

1 jalapeno pepper, deseeded and chopped

1 tablespoon apple cider vinegar

1/2 cup chicken bone broth

1/3-pound red cabbage, shredded

1 bay leaf

1 sprig rosemary

1 sprig thyme

Kitchen Equipment:

frying pan

Directions:

Cook the pork medallions in the bacon grease until they are browned on both sides.

Add the remaining ingredients and reduce the heat to medium-low. Let it cook for 13 minutes more, gently stirring periodically to ensure even cooking. Taste and adjust the seasonings.

Nutrition:

Calories 528

Fat 31.8g

Protein 51.2g

3. FESTIVE MEATLOAF

Preparation Time: 1 hour

Cooking Time: 50 minutes

Servings: 2

Ingredients:

1/4-pound ground pork

1/2-pound ground chuck

2 eggs, beaten

1/4 cup flaxseed meal

1 shallot, chopped

2 garlic cloves, minced

1/2 teaspoon smoked paprika

1/4 teaspoon dried basil

1/4 teaspoon ground cumin

Kosher salt, to taste

1/2 cup tomato puree

1 teaspoon mustard

1 teaspoon liquid monk fruit

Kitchen Equipment:

2 mixing bowl

loaf pan

oven

Directions:

In a bowl, mix thoroughly the ground meat, eggs, flaxseed meal, shallot, garlic, and spices.

In another bowl, mix the tomato puree with the mustard and liquid monk fruit, whisk to combine well.

Press the mixture into the loaf pan—Bake in the preheated oven at 360 degrees F for 30 minutes.

Nutrition: Calories 517 - **Fat** 32.3g - **Protein** 48.5g

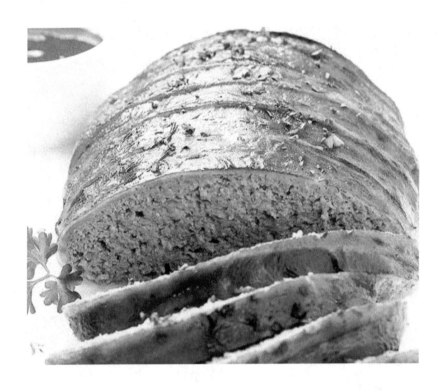

4. RICH WINTER BEEF STEW

Preparation Time: 45 minutes

Cooking Time: 50 minutes

Servings: 2

Ingredients:

1-ounce bacon, diced

3/4-pound well-marbled beef chuck, boneless and cut into 1-1/2-inch pieces

1 red bell pepper, chopped

1 green bell pepper, chopped

2 garlic cloves, minced

1/2 cup leeks, chopped

1 parsnip, chopped

Sea salt, to taste

1/4 teaspoon mixed peppercorns, freshly cracked

2 cups of chicken bone broth

1 tomato, pureed

2 cups kale, torn into pieces

1 tablespoon fresh cilantro, roughly chopped

Kitchen Equipment:

Dutch pot

Directions:

Heat a Dutch pot over medium-high flame. Now, cook the bacon until it is well browned and crisp; reserve. Then, cook the beef pieces for 3 to 5 minutes or until just browned on all sides; reserve. After that, sauté the peppers, garlic, leeks, and parsnip in the pan drippings until they are just tender and aromatic. Add the salt, peppercorns, chicken bone broth, tomato, and reserved beef to the pot. Bring to a boil. Stir in the kale leaves and continue simmering until the leaves have wilted or 3 to 4 minutes more.

Ladle into individual bowls and serve garnished with fresh cilantro and the reserved bacon.

Nutrition: - Calories 359 - **Fat** 17.8g - **Fiber** 1g

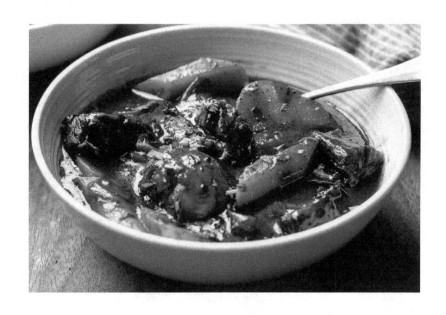

5. MINI MEATLOAVES WITH SPINACH

Preparation Time: 35 minutes

Cooking Time: 40 minutes

Servings: 2

Ingredients:

1/2-pound lean ground beef

2 tablespoons tomato paste

1 teaspoon Dijon mustard

1 egg, beaten

1/2 teaspoon ginger garlic paste

1/2 cup shallots, finely chopped

1 tablespoon canola oil

1/2 teaspoon coconut amino

1/4 cup almond meal

1 bunch spinach, chopped

1 teaspoon dried parsley flakes

1/2 teaspoon dried basil

1/2 teaspoon dried rosemary

1/2 teaspoon dried sage

1/4 teaspoon cayenne pepper

Kosher salt and ground black pepper

2 tablespoons sour cream

Kitchen Equipment:

muffin tin

oven

Directions:

Place the meat mixture into a lightly greased muffin tin. Bake the mini meatloaves in the preheated oven at 360 degrees F for 20 to 28 minutes.

Serve with sour cream and enjoy!

Nutrition: Calories 434 - **Fat** 29.4g - **Protein** 37.1g

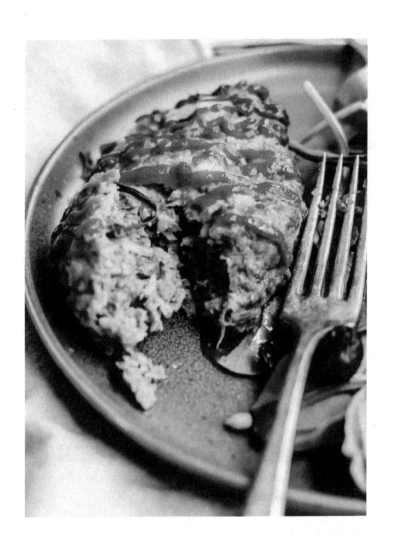

6. ZINGY LEMON FISH

Preparation Time: 50 minutes

Cooking Time: 40 minutes

Servings: 4

Ingredients:

14 ounces fresh Gurnard fish fillets

2 tablespoons lemon juice

6 tablespoons butter

½ cup fine almond flour

2 teaspoons dried chives

1 teaspoon garlic powder

2 teaspoons dried dill

2 teaspoons onion powder

Salt and pepper to taste

Kitchen Equipment:

large plate

large pan

Directions:

Add almond flour, dried herbs, salt, and spices on a large plate and stir until well combined. Spread it all over the plate evenly.

Place a large pan over medium-high heat. Add half the butter and half the lemon juice. When butter just melts, place fillets on the pan and cook for 3 minutes. Move the fillets around the pan so that it absorbs the butter and lemon juice.

Add remaining half butter and lemon juice. When butter melts, flip sides and cook the other side for 3 minutes. Serve fillets with any butter remaining in the pan.

Nutrition: Calories 406 - **Fat** 30.3g - **Protein** 29g

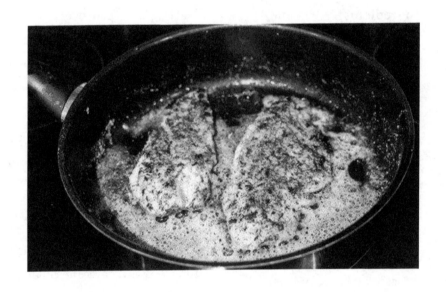

7. CREAMY KETO FISH CASSEROLE

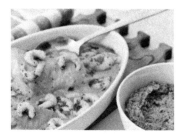

Preparation Time: 40 minutes

Cooking Time: 50 minutes

Servings: 4

Ingredients:

25 ounces of white fish (slice into bite-sized pieces)

15 ounces broccoli (small florets)

3 ounces butter + extra

6 scallions (finely chopped)

1 1/4 cups heavy whipping cream

2 tablespoons small capers

1 tablespoon dried parsley

1 tablespoon Dijon mustard

1/4 teaspoon black pepper (ground)

1 teaspoon salt

2 tablespoons olive oil

5 ounces leafy greens (finely chopped), for garnishing

Kitchen Equipment:

oven

saucepan

baking tray

Directions:

Preheat the oven to 400 degrees Fahrenheit. Cook the oil in a saucepan over medium-high heat.

Fry the broccoli florets in the hot oil for 5 minutes until tender and golden.

Transfer the fried florets to a small bowl and season it with salt and pepper. Toss the contents to ensure all the florets get an equal amount of seasoning.

Add the chopped scallions and capers to the same saucepan and fry for 2 minutes. Return the florets to the pan and mix well.

Grease a baking tray with a little amount of butter and spread the fried veggies (broccoli, scallions, and capers) in the baking tray.

Add the sliced fish to the tray and nestle it among the veggies.

Mix the heavy cream, mustard, and parsley in a small bowl and pour this mixture over the fish-veggie mixture. Top this with the remaining butter and spread gently over the contents using a spatula. Transfer to a plate and garnish with chopped greens. Serve warm and enjoy!

Nutrition: Calories 822 - Fat 69g - Protein 41g

8. KETO FISH CASSEROLE WITH MUSHROOMS AND FRENCH MUSTARD

Preparation Time: 40 minutes

Cooking Time: 50 minutes

Servings: 6

Ingredients:

25 ounces of white fish

15 ounces mushrooms (cut into wedges)

20 ounces cauliflower (cut into florets)

2 cups heavy whipping cream

3 ounces butter

2 tablespoons Dijon mustard

3 ounces olive oil

8 ounces cheese (shredded)

2 tablespoons fresh parsley

Salt & pepper, to taste

Kitchen Equipment:

oven

saucepan

Directions:

Prepare the oven to 350 degrees Fahrenheit Fry the mushroom for 5 minutes until tender and soft. Add the parsley, salt, and pepper to the mushrooms as you continue to mix well. Reduce the heat and add the mustard and heavy whipping cream to the mushroom.

Allow it simmer for 10 minutes until the sauce thickens and reduces a bit. Season the fish slices with pepper and salt. Set aside.

Sprinkle 3/4th of the cheese over the fish slices and spread the creamy mushroom over the top. Now again, top it with the remaining cheese.

Boil the cauliflower florets in lightly salted water for 5 minutes and strain the water. Place the strained florets in a bowl and add the olive oil. Mash thoroughly with a fork until you get a coarse texture—season with salt and pepper. Mix well.

Nutrition: Calories 828 - **Fat** 71g - **Protein** 39g

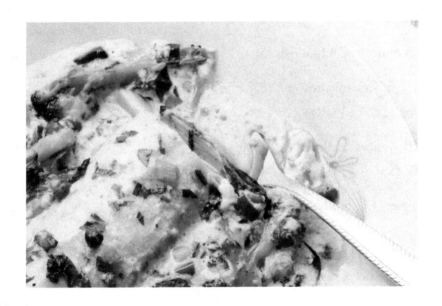

9. KETO THAI FISH WITH CURRY AND COCONUT

Preparation Time: 50 minutes

Cooking Time: 40 minutes

Servings: 4

Ingredients:

25 ounces salmon (slice into bite-sized pieces)

15 ounces cauliflower (bite-sized florets)

14 ounces coconut cream

1-ounce olive oil

4 tablespoons butter

Salt and pepper, to taste

Kitchen Equipment:

oven

Directions:

Prepare the oven to 400 degrees Fahrenheit Sprinkle salt and pepper over the salmon generously. Toss it once, if possible. Place the butter generously over all the salmon pieces and set aside.

Pour this cream mixture over the fish in the baking tray. Meanwhile, boil the cauliflower florets in salted water for 5 minutes, strain and mash the florets coarsely. Set aside. Transfer the creamy fish to a plate and serve with mashed cauliflower. Enjoy!

Nutrition:

Calories 880

Fat 75g

Protein 42g

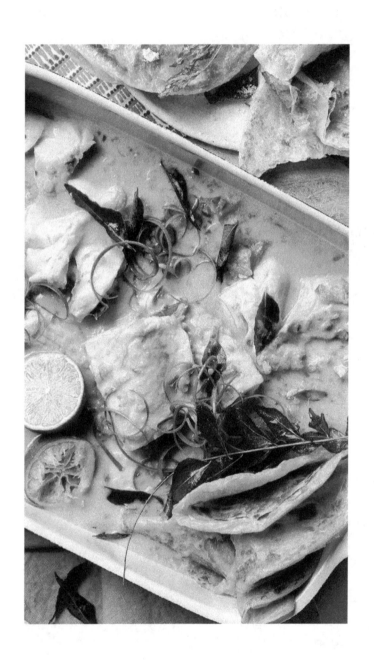

10. KETO SALMON TANDOORI WITH CUCUMBER SAUCE

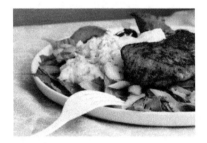

Preparation Time: 10 minutes

Cooking Time: 50 minutes

Servings: 4

Ingredients

25 ounces salmon (bite-sized pieces)

2 tablespoons coconut oil

1 tablespoon tandoori seasoning

For the cucumber sauce

1/2 shredded cucumber (squeeze out the water completely)

Juice of 1/2 lime

2 minced garlic cloves

1 1/4 cups sour cream or mayonnaise

1/2 teaspoon salt (optional)

For the crispy salad

3 1/2 ounces lettuce (torn)

3 scallions (finely chopped)

2 avocados (cubed)

1 yellow bell pepper (diced)

Juice of 1 lime

Kitchen Equipment:

oven

2 small bowl

Directions:

Preheat the oven to 350 degrees Fahrenheit Mix the tandoori seasoning with oil in a small bowl and coat the salmon pieces with this mixture. Bake for 20 minutes until soft and the salmon flakes with a fork

Take another bowl and place the shredded cucumber in it. Add the mayonnaise, minced garlic, and salt (if the mayonnaise doesn't have salt) to the shredded cucumber.

Mix the lettuce, scallions, avocados, and bell pepper in another bowl. Drizzle the contents with the lime juice.

Transfer the veggie salad to a plate and place the baked salmon over it. Top the veggies and salmon with cucumber sauce. Serve immediately and enjoy!

Nutrition: Calories 847 - **Fat** 73g - **Protein** 35g

11. MOCHA CRUNCH OATMEAL

Preparation Time: 15 minutes

Cooking Time: 5 minutes

Servings: 4

Ingredients:

1 cup of steel-cut oats

1 1/2 cup of cocoa powder

1 cup of cinnamon

1/4 teaspoon salt

2 cups of sugar

1/4 cup of agave nectar roasted mixed nuts

1/4 cup of bittersweet chocolate chips Milk or cream to serve.

Kitchen Equipment: saucepan

Directions:

Bring water to a boil. Stir in oats, cocoa powder, espresso, and salt. Bring to a boil again and raising heat to medium-low. Simmer uncovered for 20 to 30 minutes, frequently stirring until the oats hit the tenderness you need. Remove from heat and whisk in sugar or agave nectar.

While the oatmeal cooks, the mixed nuts and chocolate chips roughly chop. Place them in a small bowl to eat.

Serve with hot milk or cream on the side when the oatmeal is full, and sprinkle liberally with a coating of nut and chocolate.

Nutrition: calories 118 - **fat** 12g - **protein** 26g

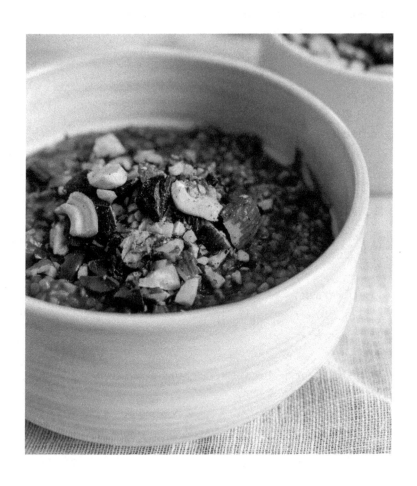

12. KETO PANCAKES

Preparation Time: 5 minutes

Cooking Time: 15 minutes

Servings: 10

Ingredients:

1/2 c. almond flour

4 oz. cream cheese softened

Four large eggs

1 tsp. lemon zest

Butter, for frying and serving

Kitchen Equipment:

nonstick skillet

Directions:

Whisk almond flour, cream cheese, eggs, and lemon zest together in a medium bowl until smooth.

Heat one tablespoon butter over medium flame in a non-stick skillet. Pour in the batter for about three tablespoons, and cook for 2 minutes until golden. Flip over and cook for 2 minutes. Switch to a plate, and start with the batter remaining.

Serve with butter on top.

Nutrition:

calories 110

fats 10g

protein 28g

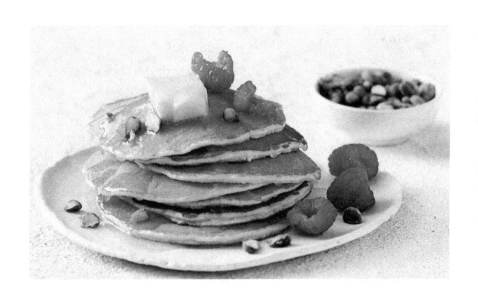

13. GREEK YOGURT FLUFFY WAFFLES

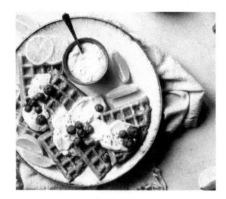

Preparation Time: 10 minutes

Cooking Time: 15 minutes

Servings: 5

Ingredients:

For the waffles:

1 cup Greek yogurt*

2 eggs whisked

2 tablespoons maple syrup

1 teaspoon vanilla extract

1 cup tapioca flour

1 cup almond flour

1 teaspoon baking powder

pinch of salt

For the toppings:

1/4 cup Greek yogurt*

1 tablespoon maple syrup

1/4 cup blueberries

1/4 cup blackberries

1/4 cup strawberries, diced

1/4 cup raspberries

Kitchen Equipment:

medium bowl

large bowl

scooper

Waffle iron

Directions:

Heat up waffle iron and oil it up. Whisk milk, eggs, maple syrup, yogurt, and the vanilla extract together in a medium bowl. Whisk the tapioca and almond flour, baking powder and salt together in a larger bowl. Add wet ingredients into dry elements and mix until well mixed.

Use an ice cream scoop to scoop in the greased waffle iron around

¼ cup of the batter and cook the waffle until it is cooked through inside and crispy outside. The batter will make roughly five-round waffles.

Once the waffles are fried, whisk the yogurt and the maple syrup together and cover each waffle with a spoonful of fruit on top!

Nutrition: **Calories** 120 - **Fats** 14g - **Protein** 31g

14. LIGHT AND CRISPY VANILLA PROTEIN WAFFLES

Preparation Time: 10 minutes

Cooking Time: 30 minutes

Servings: 4

Ingredients:

3/4 cup applesauce

4 eggs whisked

1 teaspoon vanilla extract

2 tablespoons coconut oil, melted

1 cup tapioca flour (or arrowroot powder)

1 cup Vanilla Primal Fuel protein

1 teaspoon baking soda

1/4 teaspoon cinnamon

pinch of salt

maple syrup, to garnish

coconut whipped cream, to garnish

Kitchen Equipment:

waffle iron

Directions:

Whisk applesauce, milk, vanilla extract, and coconut oil together.

Add flour and whisk the tapioca until mixed. Then add protein powder to combine and whisk again. Eventually, add cinnamon, baking soda, and a pinch of salt and blend well.

Pour batter into the waffle iron and cook until crispy. It was taking less than 5 minutes for each waffle. Repeat with batter's rest.

Garnish with cream and maple syrup, whipped with coconut.

Nutrition: calories 117 - **fats** 9g - **protein** 27g

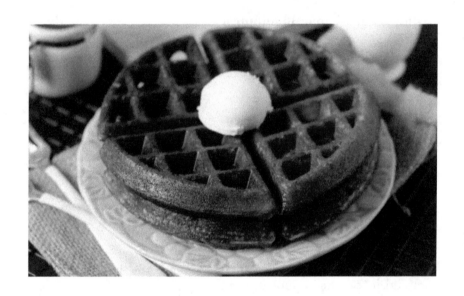

15. KETO SAUSAGE BREAKFAST SANDWICH

Preparation Time: 5 minutes

Cooking Time: 15 minutes

Servings: 3

Ingredients:

6 large eggs

2 tbsp. heavy cream

Pinch red pepper flakes

Kosher salt

Freshly ground black pepper

1 tbsp. butter

3 slices cheddar

6 frozen sausage patties, heated according to package instructions

Avocado, sliced

Kitchen Equipment:

small bowl, nonstick container

Directions:

Beat the eggs, heavy cream, and red pepper flakes together in a small bowl.

Heat butter in a non-stick container over medium flame. Pour 1/3 of the eggs into your skillet. Place a cheese slice in the center and allow it to sit for about 1 minute. Fold the egg sides in the middle, covering the cheese. Remove from saucepan and repeat with eggs left over.

Serve the eggs with avocado in between two sausage patties.

Nutrition: **Calories** 113 - **Fats** 10g - **Protein** 27g

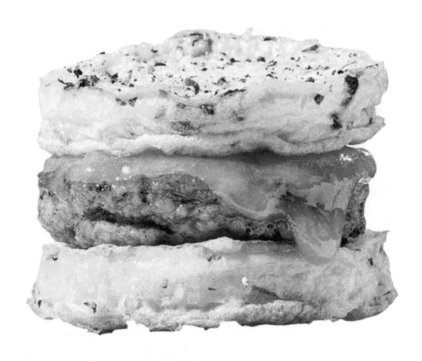

16. CABBAGE HASH BROWNS

Preparation Time: 10 minutes

Cooking Time: 25 minutes

Servings: 2

Ingredients:

2 large eggs

1/2 tsp. garlic powder

1/2 tsp. kosher salt

Freshly ground black pepper

2 c. shredded cabbage

1/4 small yellow onion, thinly sliced

1 tbsp. vegetable oil

Kitchen Equipment:

large bowl

blender

large skillet

spatula

Directions:

Whisk shells, eggs, garlic powder, and salt together in a large bowl. Season with black potatoes. Add the chicken and onion to the mixture of the eggs and blend together.

Cook oil in a large skillet over medium to high heat. In the pan, divide the mixture into four patties and press to flatten with the spatula. Cook side, until golden and tender.

Nutrition: **Calories** 109 - **Fats** 9g - **Protein** 21g

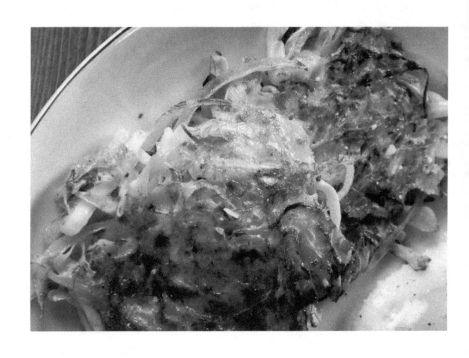

17. KETO BREAKFAST CUPS

Preparation Time: 15 minutes

Cooking Time: 40 minutes

Servings: 12

Ingredients:

2 lb. ground pork

1 tbsp. freshly chopped thyme

2 cloves garlic, minced

1/2 tsp. paprika

1/2 tsp. ground cumin

1 tsp. kosher salt

Freshly ground black pepper

2 1/2 c. chopped fresh spinach

1 c. shredded white cheddar

12 eggs

1 tbsp. freshly chopped chives

Kitchen Equipment:

oven

muffin tin

Directions:

Oven preheats to 400 ° c. combine the soiled pork, thyme, garlic, paprika, cumin, and salt in a large bowl. Season with peppers.

Attach a small handful of pork to each tin of muffin well then press the sides to make a cup. Spinach and cheese should be evenly divided between cups. Season with salt and pepper and crack an egg on top of each cup.

Bake for about 25 minutes, until eggs are set, and sausage is cooked through. Garnish and serve with chives.

Nutrition: Calories 117 - **Fat** 14g - **Protein** 30g

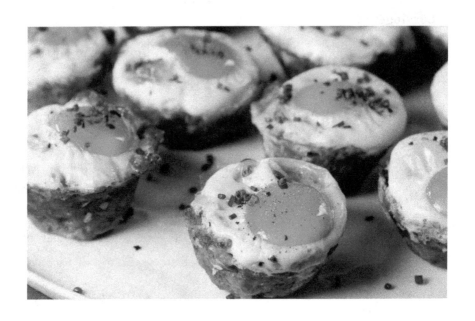

18. EGG SALAD

Preparation Time: 15 minutes

Cooking Time: 20 minutes

Servings: 6

Ingredients:

3 tbsp. mayonnaise

3 tbsp. Greek yogurt

2 tbsp. red wine vinegar

Kosher salt

Freshly ground black pepper

8 hard-boiled eggs, cut into eight pieces

8 strips bacon, cooked and crumbled

1 avocado, thinly sliced

1/2 c. crumbled blue cheese

1/2 c. cherry tomatoes

2 tbsp. freshly chopped chives

Kitchen Equipment:

small bowl

large bowl

Directions:

Stir mayonnaise, cream, and the red wine vinegar in a small bowl. Season with pepper and salt.

Kindly combine the eggs, bacon, avocado, blue cheese, and cherry tomatoes in a large serving bowl. Gradually fold in the mayonnaise dressing until the ingredients are coated slightly, then season with salt and pepper. Garnish with the chives and extra toppings.

Nutrition: **Calories** 110 - **Fats** 10g - **Protein** 26g

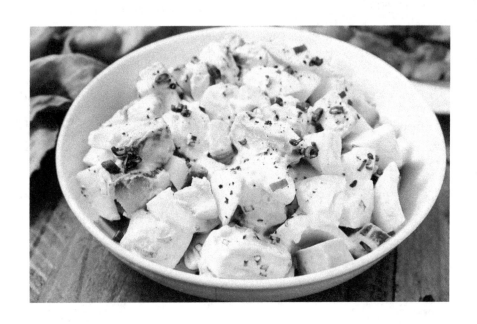

19. TACO STUFFED AVOCADOS

Preparation Time: 10 minutes

Cooking Time: 25 minutes

Servings: 8

Ingredients:

4ripe avocados

Juice of 1 lime

1 tbsp. extra-virgin olive oil

1medium onion, chopped

1 lb. ground beef

1 packet taco seasoning

Kosher salt

Freshly ground black pepper

2/3 c. shredded Mexican cheese

1/2 c. shredded lettuce

1/2 c. quartered grape tomatoes

Sour cream, for topping

Kitchen Equipment:

medium skillet

Directions:

Half and the pit avocados. Scoop a bit of avocado out using a spoon, creating a bigger well. Dice have removed avocado and set aside for later use. Squeeze lime juice (to avoid browning!) overall avocados.

Heat oil in a medium-sized skillet over medium heat. Add onion, and cook for about 5 minutes, until tender. Attach ground beef and taco seasoning, with a wooden spoon breaking up the meat. Season well and cook for about 6 minutes until the beef is no longer pink. Take off heat and drain fat.

Fill every half of the avocado with beef, then top with reserved avocado, cheese, lettuce, tomato, and a sour dollop cream.

Nutrition: Calories 107 - **Fat** 11g - **Protein** 30g

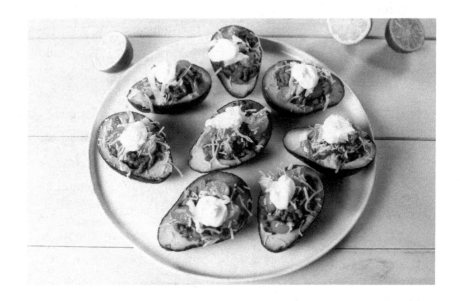

20. BUFFALO SHRIMP LETTUCE WRAPS

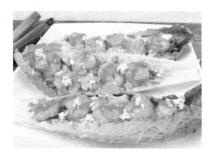

Preparation Time: 15 minutes

Cooking Time: 20 minutes

Servings: 4

Ingredients:

1/4 tbsp. butter

2 garlic cloves, minced

1/4 c. hot sauce, such as Frank's

1 tbsp. extra-virgin olive oil

1 lb. shrimp, peeled and deveined, tails removed

Kosher salt

Freshly ground black pepper

1 head romaine leaf separated, for serving

1/4 red onion, finely chopped

1 rib celery, sliced thin

1/2 c. blue cheese, crumbled

Kitchen Equipment:

saucepan

large skillet

Directions:

Make buffalo sauce: melt butter over medium heat in a small saucepan. When completely melted, add the garlic and cook for 1 minute until it is fragrant. Attach hot sauce to combine, and stir. Switch heat to low while the shrimp are cooking.

Make shrimp: heat oil in a large skillet over medium heat. Add shrimp, and add salt and pepper to season. Cook, flipping halfway, till both sides are pink and opaque, around 2 minutes per side turn off the heat and apply the sauce to the buffalo, tossing to coat.

Assemble wraps: add a small scoop of shrimp to a roman leaf center, then top with red onion, celery, and blue cheese.

Nutrition: **Calories** 108 - **Fats** 8g - **Protein** 26g

21. BROCCOLI BACON SALAD

Preparation Time: 15 minutes

Cooking Time: 15 minutes

Servings: 6

Ingredients:

For the salad:

kosher salt 3

heads broccoli, cut into bite-size pieces

Two carrots, shredded

1/2 red onion, thinly sliced

1/2 c. dried cranberries

1/2 c. sliced almonds

6 slices bacon, cooked and crumbled

For the dressing:

1/2 c. mayonnaise

3 tbsp. apple cider vinegar

kosher salt

Freshly ground black pepper

Kitchen Equipment:

medium sauce pan

large bowl

colander

Directions:

Bring 4 cups of salted water up to a boil in a medium saucepan. Prepare a large bowl of ice water while waiting for the water to boil.

Add broccoli florets to the heated water, and cook for 1 to 2 minutes until tender. Remove with a slotted spoon and put the ice water in the prepared cup. Drain flourishes within a colander when cold.

Combine broccoli, red onion, carrots, cranberries, nuts, and bacon in a large bowl. Whisk vinegar and mayonnaise together in a medium bowl and season with salt and pepper. Pour the broccoli mixture over the dressing and stir to combine.

Nutrition: **Calories** 116   -
Fats 12g - **Protein** 37g

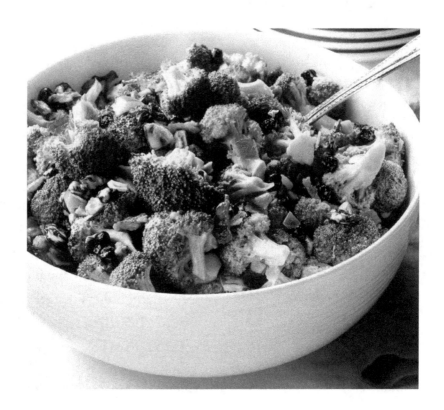

22. KETO SALAD

Preparation Time: 15 minutes

Cooking Time: 15 minutes

Servings: 4

Ingredients:

3 tbsp. mayonnaise

2 tsp. lemon juice

1 tbsp. finely chopped chives

Freshly ground black pepper

Kosher salt

6 hard-boiled eggs, peeled and chopped

1 avocado, cubed

Lettuce, for serving

Cooked bacon, for serving

Kitchen Equipment:

medium bowl

Directions:

Whisk the mayonnaise, lemon juice, and chives together in a medium bowl. Season with pepper and salt. Add eggs and avocado to mix and throw gently. Serve with Bacon and Lettuce.

Nutrition:

Calories 114 - **Fat** 9g - **Protein** 30g

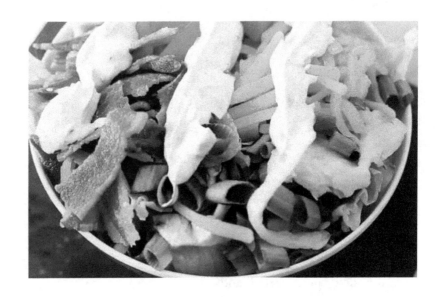

23.KETO BACON SUSHI

Preparation Time: 10 minutes

Cooking Time: 30 minutes

Servings: 12

Ingredients:

6 slices bacon halved

2 Persian cucumbers, thinly sliced

2 medium carrots, thinly sliced

1 avocado, sliced

4 oz. cream cheese softened

Sesame seeds, for garnish

Kitchen Equipment:

oven

aluminum foil

baking sheet

Directions:

Preheat oven to around 400o. Strip an aluminum foil baking sheet and fit it with a refrigerating rack. Lay the bacon halves in an even layer and bake for 11 to 13 minutes, until slightly crisp yet pliable. In the meantime, the cucumbers, carrots, and avocado are sliced into parts around the bacon width.

Place one even layer of cream cheese on each slice when the bacon is cool enough to touch. Equally, divide vegetables between the bacon and put them on one end. Roll up tightly on vegetables.

Garnish, and serve with sesame seeds

Nutrition: Calories 109 - **Fat** 10g - **Protein** 27g

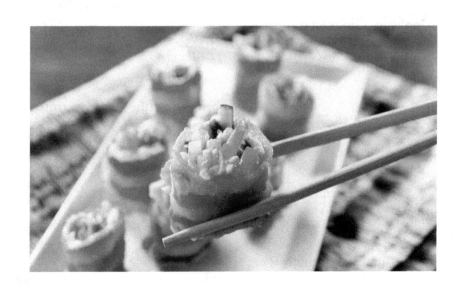

24. LOADED CAULIFLOWER SALAD

Preparation Time: 10 minutes

Cooking Time: 30 minutes

Servings: 6

Ingredients:

1 large head cauliflower, cut into florets

6 slices bacon

1/2 c. sour cream

1/4 c. mayonnaise

1 tbsp. lemon juice

1/2 tsp. garlic powder

Kosher salt

Freshly ground black pepper

1 1/2 c. shredded cheddar

1/4 c. finely chopped chives

Kitchen Equipment:

large skillet

Directions:

Bring around ¼ cup of water into a large skillet to boil. Add cauliflower, cover pan and steam for about 4 minutes, until tender. Drain and allow to cool while preparing other ingredients.

Start cooking the pork in a pan over medium heat, around 3 minutes per side, until crispy. Switch to a towel-lined sheet of paper for drain, then cut.

Whisk the sour cream, mayonnaise, lemon juice, and garlic powder together in a big bowl. Remove cauliflower and gently toss. Add salt and pepper, then fold into bacon, cheddar, and chives. Serve warm, or at ambient temperature.

Nutrition: Calories 440 - **Fat** 135g - **Protein** 26g

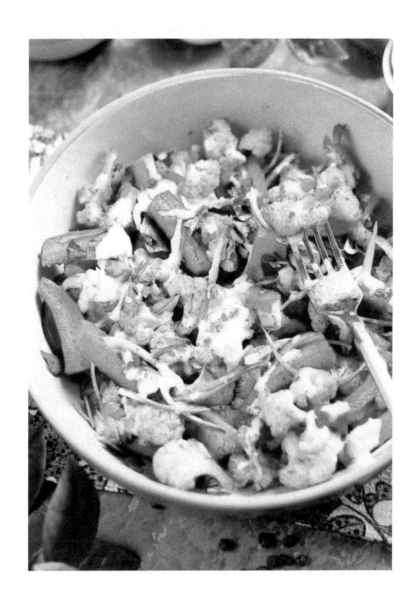

25. CAPRESE ZOODLES

Preparation Time: 10 minutes

Cooking Time: 25 minutes

Servings: 4

Ingredients:

4 large zucchinis

2 tbsp. extra-virgin olive oil

kosher salt

Freshly ground black pepper

2 c. cherry tomatoes halved

1 c. mozzarella balls, quartered if large

1/4 c. fresh basil leaves

2 tbsp. balsamic vinegar

Kitchen Equipment:

spiralizer

large bowl

Directions:

Creating zoodles out of zucchini using a spiralizer. In a large bowl, add the zoodles, mix with the olive oil and season with the salt and pepper. Let them marinate for 15 minutes.

In zoodles, add the tomatoes, mozzarella, and basil and toss until combined. Drizzle, and drink with balsamic.

Nutrition: - **Calories** 116 - **Fat** 115g - **Protein** 31g

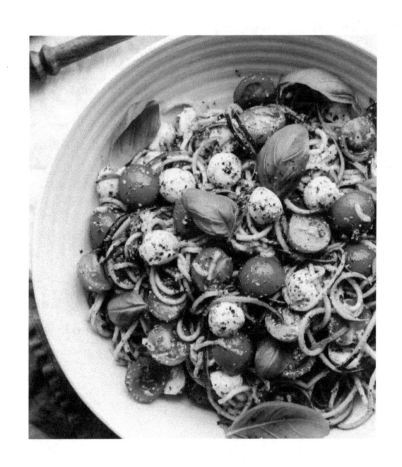

26. CHICKEN SPINACH CURRY

Preparation Time: 10 minutes

Cooking Time: 17 minutes

Servings: 4

Ingredients:

2 tomatoes, chopped

4 ounces spinach, chopped

1/3-pound curry paste

1 1/2 cups yogurt

4 pounds chicken, cubed

1 tablespoon olive oil

1 onion, cut to make slices

1 tablespoon chopped coriander

Kitchen Equipment:

mixing bowl

instant pot

Directions:

Combine the chicken, curry paste, and yogurt in a mixing bowl. Wrap and soak in the fridge for 30 minutes. Situate the Instant Pot over a dry surface in your kitchen. Open and turn it on.

Click "SAUTE" cooking function; pour the oil in it and allow it to heat. In the pot, stir in the onions; cook (while stirring) until turns translucent and softened. Mix the tomatoes and cook for another minute.

Pour the chicken mixture, mix in the spinach and coriander; gently stir to mix well. Close the lid. Select "MANUAL" cooking function; timer to 15 minutes with default "HIGH" pressure mode.

Let the pressure to build to cook the ingredients. After cooking time is over click "CANCEL". Set "QPR" cooking function.

This setting is for quick release of inside pressure.

Gradually open the lid, put the cooked dish in the serving plates.

Nutrition:

Calories 384   -   **Fat** 18g   -   **Protein** 12g

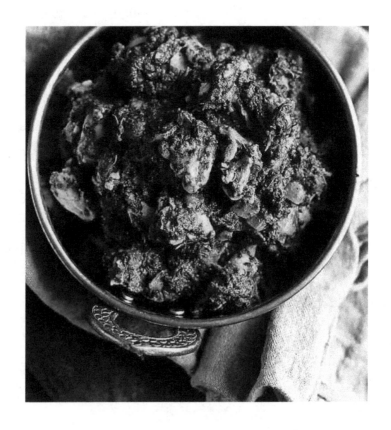

27. SUPER HERBED FISH

Preparation Time: 10 minutes

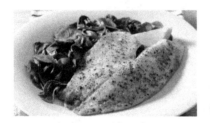

Cooking Time: 6 minutes

Servings: 1

Ingredients:

1 tablespoon chopped basil

2 teaspoons lime zest

1 tablespoon lime juice

1 tablespoon olive oil

1 4-ounce fish fillet

1 rosemary sprig

1 thyme sprig

1 teaspoon Dijon mustard

¼ teaspoon garlic powder

Pinch of salt

Pinch of pepper

1 ½ cups water

Kitchen Equipment:

parchment paper

mixing bowl

aluminum foil

instant pot

Directions:

Season the fish with salt and paper. Wrap a piece of parchment paper and sprinkle with zest. Whisk together the oil, juice, and mustard in a mixing bowl and brush over. Top with the herbs. Wrap the fish with the parchment paper. Wrap the wrapped fish in an aluminum foil. Get the Instant Pot in platform in your kitchen. Open and switch it on. In the pot, pour water. Arrange a trivet or steamer basket inside that came with Instant Pot. Now place/ arrange the foil over the trivet/ basket.

Close the lid.

Press "MANUAL" cooking function; timer to 5 minutes with

default "HIGH" pressure mode. Let the pressure to build to cook the ingredients.

After cooking time is over select "CANCEL". Adjust to "QPR" cooking function. For fast release of inside pressure. Lightly open the lid, take out the cooked recipe in serving bowls.

Nutrition: Calories 246 - Fat 9g - Carbohydrates 1g

28. TURKEY AVOCADO CHILI

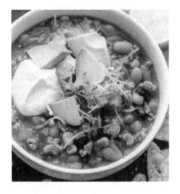

Preparation Time: 10 minutes

Cooking Time: 50 minutes

Servings: 4

Ingredients:

2 ½ pounds lean (finely ground) turkey

2 cups diced tomatoes

2-ounce tomato paste, sugar-free

1 tablespoon olive oil

½ chopped large yellow onion

8 minced garlic cloves

1 (4-ounce) can green chilies with liquid

2 tablespoons Worcestershire sauce

1 tablespoon dried oregano

¼ cup red chili powder

2 tablespoons (finely ground) cumin

Salt and freshly (finely ground) black pepper, as per taste preference

1 pitted and sliced avocado, peeled

Kitchen Equipment:

Instant pot

Directions:

Place the Instant Pot over a dry podium in your kitchen. Switch it on.

Select "SAUTE" cooking function; fill the oil in it and allow it to heat.

In the pot, mix the onions; cook (while stirring) until turns translucent and softened for around 4-5 minutes.

Add the garlic and cook for about 1 minute.

Add the turkey and cook for about 8-9 minutes. Stir in remaining ingredients except for the avocado.

Close the lid.

Choose "MEAT/STEW" cooking function; timer to 35 minutes with default "HIGH" pressure mode.

Allow the pressure to build to cook the ingredients.

After cooking time is over click "CANCEL". Set to "NPR" cooking function for the natural release, and it takes around 10 minutes to release pressure slowly.

Gradually open the lid, pull out the cooked dish and place in serving plates, top with the avocado slices, and enjoy the Keto recipe.

Nutrition: Calories 346 - **Fat** 19g - **Fiber** 5g

29. CHEESY TOMATO SHRIMP

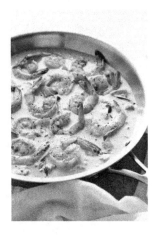

Preparation Time: 10 minutes

Cooking Time: 15 minutes

Servings: 4

Ingredients:

2 tablespoons olive oil

½ cup veggie broth

¼ cup chopped cilantro

2 tablespoons lime juice

1 ½ pounds shrimp, peeled and deveined

1 ½ pounds tomatoes, chopped

1 jalapeno, diced

1 onion, diced

1 cup shredded cheddar cheese

1 teaspoon minced garlic

Kitchen Equipment:

Instant pot

Directions:

Put the Instant Pot in a surface in your kitchen. Open its top lid and turn it on. Set "SAUTE" cooking function; put the oil in it and allow it to heat. In the pot, place the onions; cook (while stirring) until turns translucent and softened for around 2-3 minutes.

Add garlic and sauté for 30-60 seconds. Stir in the broth, cilantro, and tomatoes and secure the lid

Find and press "MANUAL" cooking function; timer to 9 minutes with default "HIGH" pressure mode. Let the pressure cook the ingredients.

After cooking time is over press "CANCEL". set "NPR" cooking function for the release, for around 10 minutes to release pressure slowly.

Add the shrimps. Close the top lid. Find and press "MANUAL" cooking function; timer to 2 minutes with default "HIGH" pressure mode.

Let the pressure to build to cook the ingredients. After cooking time is over select "CANCEL". Then press "NPR" cooking function for the release of inside pressure, and for around 10 minutes to release pressure slowly.

Slowly transfer the cooked meals into serving bowls, top with the cheddar, and enjoy the Keto recipe.

Nutrition: Calories 268 - **Fat** 16g - **Carbohydrates** 7g

30. CAJUN ROSEMARY CHICKEN

Preparation Time: 10 minutes

Cooking Time: 30 minutes

Servings: 4

Ingredients:

2 teaspoons Cajun seasoning

1 lemon, halved

1 yellow onion, make quarters

1 teaspoon garlic salt

1 medium chicken

2 rosemary sprigs

1 tablespoon coconut oil

1/4 teaspoon pepper

1 1/2 cups chicken broth

Kitchen Equipment:

Instant pot

Directions:

Season the chicken and Cajun seasoning. Stuff the lemon, onion, and rosemary in the chicken's cavity. Get the Instant Pot then open its top lid and turn it on.

Press "SAUTE" cooking function; place the oil in it and allow it to heat. Put the meat; cook (while stirring) until turns evenly brown from all sides. Add the broth; gently stir to mix well.

Close the lid then click "MANUAL" cooking function; timer to 25 minutes with default "HIGH" pressure mode.

Let the pressure to build to cook the ingredients. After cooking time is over press "CANCEL". Then "NPR" cooking function for the natural release of inside pressure, and for around 10 minutes to release pressure slowly.

Gradually open the lid, place dish in serving plates or serving bowls, and enjoy the Keto recipe.

Nutrition: Calories 236 - **Fat** 26g - **Fiber** 5g

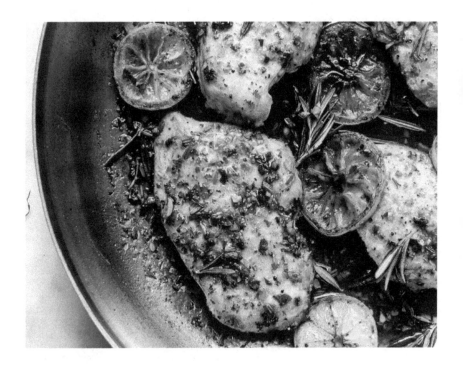

31. SRIRACHA TUNA KABOBS

Preparation Time: 4 minutes

Cooking Time: 9 minutes

Servings: 4

Ingredients

4 tablespoon Huy Fong chili garlic sauce

1 tablespoon sesame oil infused with garlic

1 tablespoon ginger, fresh, grated

1 tablespoon garlic, minced

1 red onion, cut into quarters

2 cups bell peppers, red, green, yellow

1 can whole water chestnuts

½ pound fresh mushrooms halved

32 oz. boneless tuna, chunks or steaks

1 Splenda packet

2 zucchinis, sliced

1 inch thick, keep skins on

Kitchen Equipment:

skewers

blender

griller

Directions:

Layer the tuna and the vegetable pieces evenly onto 8 skewers. Combine the spices and the oil and chili sauce, add the Splenda Quickly blend, either in a blender or by Quickly whipping.

Brush onto the kabob pieces, make sure every piece is coated Grill 4 minutes on each district, check to ensure the tuna is cooked to taste. Serving size is two skewers.

Mix the marinade ingredients and store in a covered container in the fridge. Place all the vegetables in one container in the fridge. Place the tuna in a separate zip-lock bag.

Nutrition: **Calories** 467 - **Protein** 56g - **Fiber** 3.5g

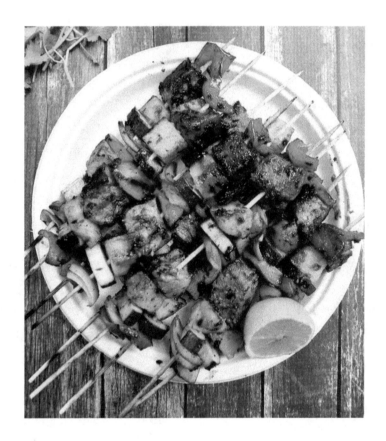

32. PORK CUTLETS WITH SPANISH ONION

Preparation Time: 15 minutes

Cooking Time: 15 minutes

Servings: 4

Ingredients:

- 1 tablespoon of olive oil

- 2 pork cutlets

- 1 bell pepper (deveined and sliced)

- 1 Spanish of onion (chopped)

- 2 garlic cloves (minced)

- 1/2 teaspoon of hot sauce

- 1/2 teaspoon of mustard

- 1/2 teaspoon of paprika

Kitchen Equipment:

- saucepan

Directions:

1. Fry the pork cutlets for 3 to 4 minutes until evenly golden and crispy on both sides.

2. Set the temperature to medium and add the bell pepper, Spanish onion, garlic, hot sauce, and mustard; continue cooking until the vegetables have softened, for a further 3 minutes.

3. Sprinkle with paprika, salt, and black pepper.

4. Serve immediately and enjoy!

Nutrition: **Calories:** 403 - **Fat:** 24.1g - **Total Carbs:** 3.4g

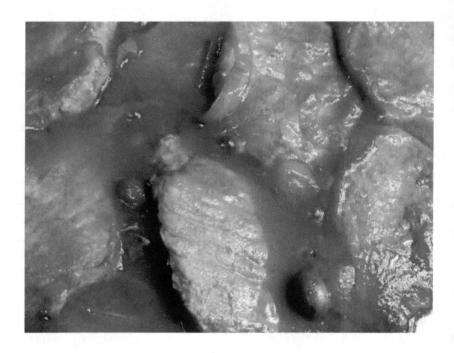

33. RICH AND EASY PORK RAGOUT

Preparation Time: 15 minutes

Cooking Time: 15 minutes

Servings: 4

Ingredients:

- 1 teaspoon of lard (melted at room temperature)

- 3/4-pound of pork butt (cut into bite-sized cubes)

- 1 red bell pepper (deveined and chopped)

- 1 poblano pepper (deveined and chopped)

- 2 cloves of garlic (pressed)

- 1/2 cup of leeks, chopped

- 1/2 teaspoon of mustard seeds

- 1/4 teaspoon of ground allspice

- 1/4 teaspoon of celery seeds

- 1 cup of roasted vegetable broth

- 2 vine-ripe tomatoes (pureed)

Kitchen Equipment:

- stockpot

Directions:

1. Melt the lard in a stockpot over moderate heat.

2. Once hot, cook the pork cubes for 4 to 6 minutes, occasionally stirring to ensure even cooking.

3. Then, stir in the vegetables and continue cooking until they are tender and fragrant.

4. Add in the salt, black pepper, mustard seeds, allspice, celery seeds,

roasted vegetable broth, and tomatoes.

5. Reduce the heat to simmer. Let it simmer for 30 minutes longer or until everything is heated through.

6. Ladle into individual bowls and serve hot. Bon appétit!

Nutrition: **Calories:** 389 - **Fat:** 24.3g - **Total Carbs:** 5.4g

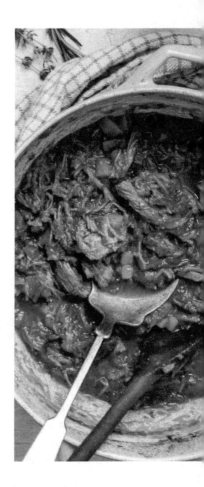

34. MELT-IN-YOUR-MOUTH PORK ROAST

Preparation Time: 35 minutes

Cooking Time: 40 minutes

Servings: 2

Ingredients:

1-pound pork shoulder

4 tablespoons red wine

1 teaspoon stone-ground mustard

1 tablespoon coconut aminos

1 tablespoon lemon juice

1 tablespoon sesame oil

2 sprigs rosemary

1 teaspoon sage

1 shallot, peeled and chopped

1/2 celery stalk, chopped

1/2 head garlic, separated into cloves

Kitchen Equipment:

ceramic dish

baking dish

Directions:

Place the pork shoulder, red wine, mustard, coconut aminos, lemon juice, sesame oil, rosemary, and sage in a ceramic dish; cover and let it marinate in your refrigerator at least 1 hour.

Discard a lightly greased baking dish. Scatter the vegetables around the pork shoulder and sprinkle with salt and black pepper. Roast in the preheated oven at 390 degrees F for 15 minutes.

Now, reduce the temperature to 310 degrees F and continue baking an additional 40 to 45 minutes. Baste the meat with the reserved marinade once or twice.

Place on cooling racks before carving and serving. Bon appétit!

Nutrition: Calories 497 - **Fat** 35g - **Protein** 40.2g

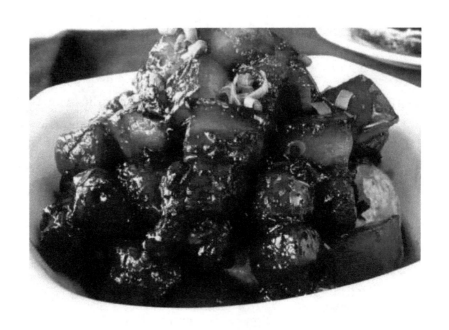

35. CHUNKY PORK SOUP WITH MUSTARD GREENS

Preparation Time: 25 minutes

Cooking Time: 30 minutes

Servings: 2

Ingredients:

1 tablespoon olive oil

1 bell pepper, deveined and chopped

2 garlic cloves, pressed

1/2 cup scallions, chopped

1/2-pound ground pork (84% lean)

1 cup beef bone broth

1 cup of water

1/2 teaspoon crushed red pepper flakes

1 bay laurel

1 teaspoon fish sauce

2 cups mustard greens, torn into pieces

1 tablespoon fresh parsley, chopped

Kitchen Equipment:

sauté pan

Directions:

Coat, once hot, sauté the pepper, garlic, and scallions until tender or about 3 minutes.

After that, stir in the ground pork and cook for 5 minutes more or until well browned, stirring periodically.

Add in the beef bone broth, water, red pepper, salt, black pepper, and bay laurel. Reduce the temperature to simmer and cook, covered, for 10 minutes. Afterward, stir in the fish sauce and mustard greens.

Remove from the heat; let it stand until the greens are wilted. Ladle into individual bowls and

serve garnished with fresh
parsley.

Nutrition: Calories 344 - **Fat**
25.g

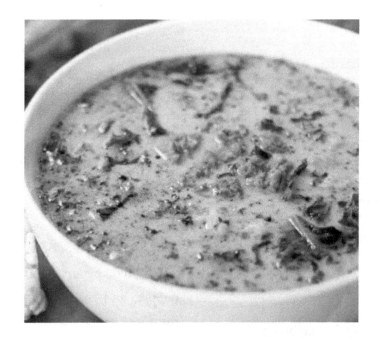

36. PULLED PORK WITH MINT AND CHEESE

Preparation Time: 20 minutes

Cooking Time: 15 minutes

Servings: 2

Ingredients:

1 teaspoon lard, melted at room temperature

3/4 pork Boston butt, sliced

2 garlic cloves, pressed

1/2 teaspoon red pepper flakes, crushed

1/2 teaspoon black peppercorns, freshly cracked

Sea salt, to taste

2 bell peppers, deveined and sliced

1 tablespoon fresh mint leave snipped

4 tablespoons cream cheese

Kitchen Equipment:

cast-iron skillet

Directions:

Melt the lard in a cast-iron skillet over a moderate flame. Once hot, brown the pork for 2 minutes per side until caramelized and crispy on the edges.

Set the temperature to medium-low and continue cooking another 4 minutes, turning over periodically. Shred the pork with two forks and return to the skillet.

Add the garlic, red pepper, black peppercorns, salt, and bell pepper and continue cooking for a further 2 minutes or until the peppers are just tender and fragrant.

Serve with fresh mint and a dollop of cream cheese. Enjoy!

Nutrition: Calories 370 - **Fat** 21.9g - **Protein:** 34.9g

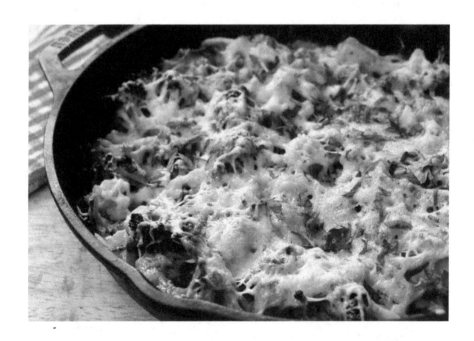

37. CHICKEN CASSEROLE

Preparation Time: 19 minutes

Cooking Time: 29 minutes

Servings: 4

Ingredients

6 Tortilla Factory low-carb whole wheat tortillas, torn into small pieces

1 ½ cups hand-shredded cheese, Mexican

1 beaten egg

1 cup milk

2 cups cooked chicken, shredded

1 can Ro-tel

½ cup salsa Verde

Kitchen Equipment:

8x8 glass baking dish

oven

Directions:

Brush an 8 x 8 glass baking dish with oil. Heat oven to 375 degrees Combine everything, but reserve ½ cup8 x 8 glass baking tray with margarine. Heat oven to 375 degrees Combine everything, but reserve ½ cup of the cheese Bake it for 29 minutes

Take it out of the furnace and add ½ cup cheese Broil for about 2 minutes to melt the cheese Let the casserole cool. Slice into 6 slices and place in freezer containers, (1 cup with a lid) Fix. Microwave for 2 minutes to serve. Top with sour cream, if desired.

Nutrition: 265 Calories - 20g **Protein** - 10g **Fiber**

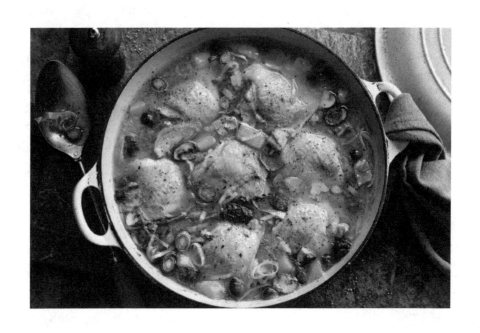

38. STEAK WITH SPICE SALAD

Preparation Time: 4 minutes

Cooking Time: 4 minutes

Servings: 2

Ingredients

2 tablespoon sriracha sauce

1 tablespoon garlic, minced

1 tablespoon ginger, fresh, grated

1 bell pepper, yellow, cut into thin strips

1 bell pepper, red, cut into thin strips

1 tablespoon sesame oil, garlic

1 Splenda packet

½ tablespoon curry powder

½ tablespoon rice wine vinegar

8 oz. of beef sirloin, cut into strips

2 cups baby spinach, stemmed

½ head butter lettuce, torn or chopped into bite-sized pieces

Kitchen Equipment:

2 bowls

Directions:

Place the garlic, sriracha sauce, 1 tablespoon sesame oil, rice wine vinegar, and Splenda into a basin and combine nicely. Pour half of this mix into a zip-lock bag. Add the steak to marinade while you are preparing the salad. Assemble the brightly colored salad by layering in two bowls.

You must put in the spinach into the bottom of the bowl. Place the butter lettuce next. Mix the two peppers and place on top.

Remove the steak from the marinade and discard the liquid and bag.

Heat the sesame oil and rapidly stir fry the steak until desired doneness, it should have about 3 minutes. Situate the steak on top of the salad.

Drizzle with the remaining dressing (another field of marinade mix). Sprinkle sriracha sauce across the salad.

Combine the salad ingredients and stand in a zip-lock bag in the fridge. Mix the marinade and halve into 2 zip-lock bags. Place the sriracha sauce into a small sealed container. Slice the steak and freeze in a zip-lock bag with the marinade. To make, mix the ingredients like the initial Directions:. Stir fry the marinated beef for 4 minutes to take into consideration the beef is frozen.

Nutrition: **Calories** 350 - **Total Fat** 23g - **Protein** 28g

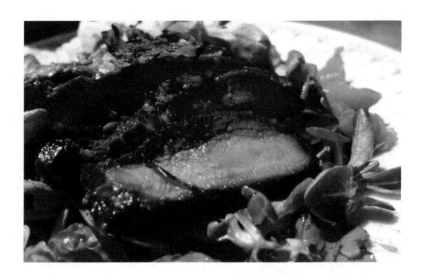

39. CHICKEN CHOW MEIN STIR FRY

Preparation Time: 9 minutes

Cooking Time: 14 minutes

Servings: 4

Ingredients

1/2 cup sliced onion

2 tablespoon Oil, sesame garlic flavored

4 cups shredded Bok-Choy

1 cup Sugar Snap Peas

1 cup fresh bean sprouts

3 stalks Celery, chopped

1 1/2 tablespoon minced Garlic

1 packet Splenda

1 cup Broth, chicken

2 tablespoon Soy Sauce

1 tablespoon ginger, freshly minced

1 tablespoon cornstarch

4 boneless Chicken Breasts, cooked/sliced thinly

Kitchen Equipment:

skillet

Directions:

Place the bok-choy, peas, celery in a skillet with 1 T garlic oil. Stir fry until bok-choy is softened to liking. Add remaining ingredients except for the cornstarch.

If too thin, stir cornstarch into ½ cup lukewarm water when smooth flow into skillet. Bring cornstarch and chow Mein to a one-minute boil. Turn off the heat source. Stir sauce then wait for 4 minutes to serve, after the chow Mein has thickened.

Freeze in covered containers. Heat for 2 minutes in the microwave before serving.

Nutrition: Calories 368 -
Total Fat 18g - Protein42g

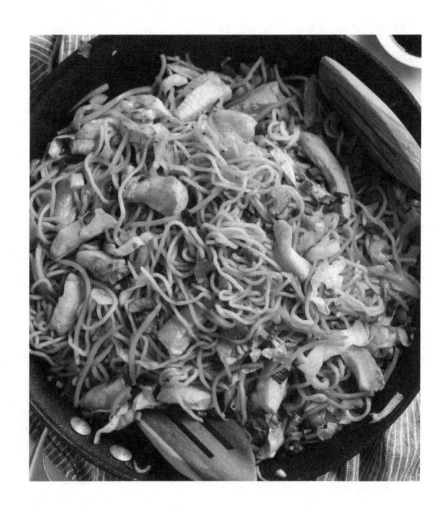

40. SALMON WITH BOK-CHOY

Preparation Time: 9 minutes

Cooking Time: 9 minutes

Servings: 4

Ingredients

1 cup red peppers, roasted, drained

2 cups chopped bok-choy

1 tablespoon salted butter

5 oz. salmon steak

1 lemon, sliced very thinly

1/8 tablespoon black pepper

1 tablespoon olive oil

2 tablespoon sriracha sauce

Kitchen Equipment:

skillet

Directions:

Place oil in a skillet Place all but 4 slices of lemon in the skillet. Place the bok choy with the black pepper.

Stir fry the bok-choy with the lemons. Remove and place on four plates. Place the butter in the skillet and stir fry the salmon, turning once.

Place the salmon on the bed of bok-choy. Split the red peppers and encircle the salmon. Transfer a slice of lemon on top of the salmon.

Drizzle with sriracha sauce. Freeze the cooked salmon in individual zip-lock bags. Place the bok-choy, with the remaining ingredients into one-cup containers. Microwave the salmon for one minute and the frozen bok choy for two. Assemble to serve.

Nutrition: Calories 410 - **Total Fat** 30g - **Protein** 30g

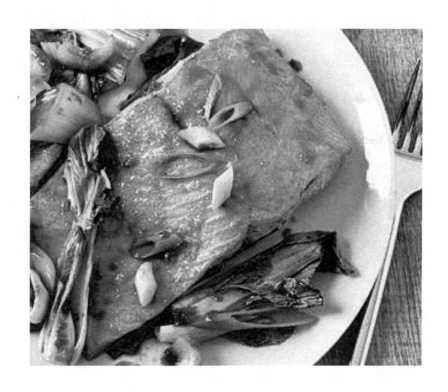

41. TORTILLA BREAKFAST CASSEROLE

Preparation Time: 10 minutes

Cooking Time: 30 minutes

Servings: 12

Ingredients

1 Pound Bacon, Cooked and Crumbled

1 Pound Pork Sausage. Cooked and Crumbled

1 Pound Package Diced Ham

10 8-inch Tortillas, Cut in half 8 Large Eggs

1 1/2 Cups Milk

1/2 Teaspoon Salt

1/2 Teaspoon Pepper

1/2 Teaspoon Garlic Powder

1/2 teaspoon Hot Sauce

2 Cups Shredded Cheddar Cheese

1 Cup Mozzarella or Monterrey Jack Cheese

Kitchen Equipment:

9x13 baking dish

pan

large bowl

oven

Directions:

Grease 9x13-inch baking dish with 2 teaspoons of butter or sprinkle with nonstick spray oil. Bake 1/3 layer of tortillas in the bottom of the pot and cover with baked bacon and 1/3 layer of cheese.

Place another third of the tortillas in the pan and cover with the cooked and chopped sausages and place another third of the cheese in layers.

Repeat with the last tortilla, ham and cheese 1/3. Mix eggs, milk, salt, pepper, garlic powder, and hot sauce. Pour the egg mixture evenly over the pot.

If desired, cover overnight and refrigerate or bake immediately. Set the oven to 350 degrees. Bake covered with foil for 45 minutes. Find and cook for another 20 minutes until the cheese is completely melted and cooked in a pan.

Nutrition: Calories 447 - Fat 32.6g - Carbohydrates 14.6g

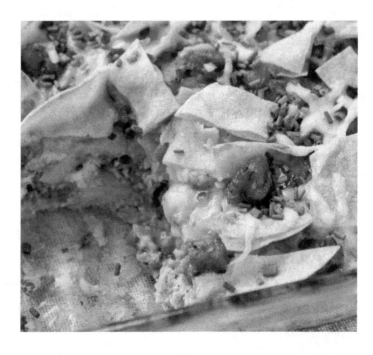

42. PECAN-BANANA POPS

Preparation Time: 10 minutes

Cooking Time: 15 minutes

Servings: 4

Ingredients

4 large just-ripe bananas

2 tablespoons raw honey

4 Popsicle sticks

3A cup chopped pecans

½ cup almond butter

Kitchen Equipment:

microwave

small bowl

baking sheet

wax paper or foil

Directions:

Peel and cut one end from each banana, and insert a Popsicle stick into the cut end.

Combine together the almond butter and honey, and heat in the microwave for 10 to 15 seconds, or just until the mixture is slightly thinned. Pour onto a sheet of wax paper or aluminum foil and spread with a spatula.

On another piece of wax paper or foil, spread the chopped pecans — Line a small baking sheet or large plate with the third piece of wax paper or foil.

Roll each banana first in the honey mixture until well coated, then in the nuts until completely covered, pressing down gently, so the nuts adhere.

Place each finished banana onto the baking sheet. When all of the bananas have been coated, place the sheet in the freezer for at least 2 hours. For long-term storage, transfer the frozen

bananas into a resealable plastic
bag.

Nutrition: Fat   14g   -
Carbohydrates   7g   -
Protein14g

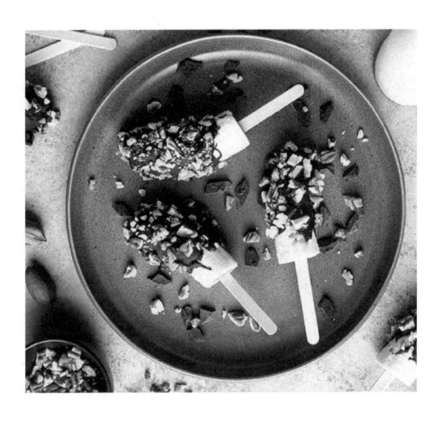

43. GREEK BREAKFAST WRAPS

Preparation Time: 10 minutes

Cooking Time: 15 minutes

Servings: 2

Ingredients

1 teaspoon olive oil

½ cup fresh baby spinach leaves

1 tablespoon fresh basil

4 egg whites, beaten

½ teaspoon salt

¼ teaspoon freshly ground black pepper

¼ cup crumbled low-fat feta cheese

2 (8-inch) whole-wheat tortillas

Kitchen Equipment:

small skillet

microwave

Directions:

Cook the olive oil over medium heat. Place the spinach and basil to the pan and sauté for about 2 minutes, or just until the spinach is wilted. Add the egg whites to the pan, season with the salt and pepper, and sauté, continue stirring until the egg whites are firm.

Turn off the heat and topped with the feta cheese. Warm up the tortillas until softened and warm in the microwave. Divide the eggs between the tortillas and wrap up burrito-style.

Nutrition: **Fat** 10.4g   - **Carbohydrate** 4.5g - **Protein** 10.6g

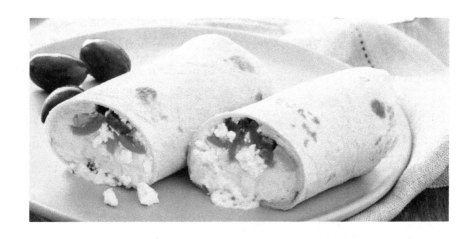

44. CURRIEDCHICKENBREAST WRAPS

Preparation Time: 10 minutes

Cooking Time: 10 minutes

Servings: 2

Ingredients

6 ounces cooked chicken breast, cubed

1 small Gala or Granny Smith apple, cored and chopped

2 tablespoons plain low-fat yogurt

1 cup spring lettuce mix or baby lettuce

1 teaspoon Dijon mustard

½ teaspoon mild curry powder

2 (8-inch) whole-wheat tortillas

Kitchen Equipment:

Small bowl

Directions:

Stir well the chicken, yogurt, Dijon mustard, and curry powder to combine. Add the apple and stir until blended.

Split the lettuce between the tortillas and top each with half of the chicken mixture. Roll up burrito-style and serve.

Nutrition:

Total fat 5g - **Carbohydrates** 18g - **Protein** 28g

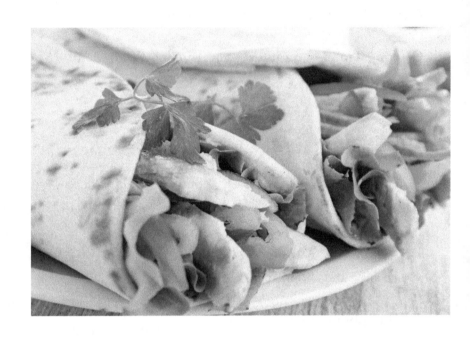

45. BAKED SALMON FILLETS WITH TOMATO AND MUSHROOMS

Preparation Time: 10 minutes

Cooking Time: 20 minutes

Servings: 2

Ingredients

2 (4-ounce) skin-on salmon fillets

2 teaspoons olive oil, divided

½ teaspoon salt

¼ teaspoon freshly ground black pepper

½ teaspoon chopped fresh dill

½ cup diced fresh tomato

½ cup sliced fresh mushrooms

Kitchen Equipment:

oven

aluminum foil

pastry brush

Directions:

Set the oven at 375 degrees and line a baking sheet with aluminum foil. You are using your fingers or a pastry brush, coat both sides of the fillets with ½ teaspoon of the olive oil each. Place the salmon skin-side down on the pan. Sprinkle salt and pepper equally all round.

In a small plate, mix the remaining 1 teaspoon olive oil, the tomato, mushrooms, and dill; stir well to combine. Spoon the mixture over the fillets.

Wrap it with foil to seal the fish, place the pan on the middle oven rack, and bake for about 20 minutes, or until the salmon flakes easily.

Nutrition: **Fat** 12.2g   -
Carbohydrate 21g   -   **Protein**
25.1g

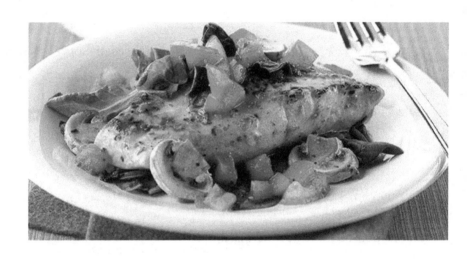

46. CINNAMON AND SPICE OVERNIGHT OATS

Preparation Time: 10 minutes

Cooking Time: 0 minute

Servings: 1

Ingredients

75g rolled oats

100ml milk

75g yogurt

1 tsp. honey

1/2 tsp. vanilla extract

1/8th tsp. Schwartz ground cinnamon

20g raisins

Kitchen Equipment:

bowl

microwave

Directions:

Incorporate all ingredients to a bowl and mix well. Cover overnight or at least one hour and refrigerate.

Exit the refrigerator or heat it in the microwave immediately or slowly.

Nutrition:

Carbohydrates 15g - **Protein** 26g - **Fat** 34g

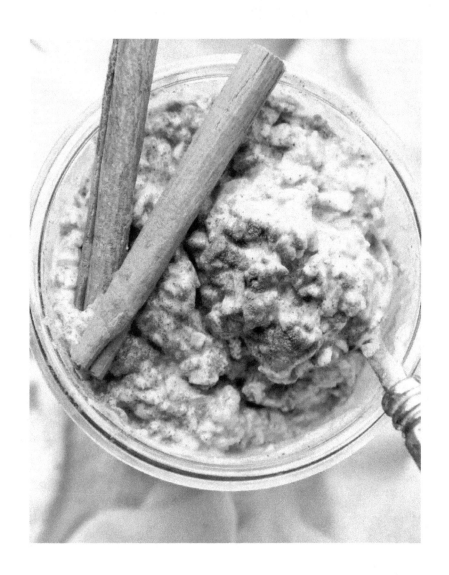

47. MEXICAN CASSEROLE

Preparation Time: 10 minutes

Cooking Time: 20 minutes

Servings: 6

Ingredients

1-pound lean ground beef

2 cups salsa

1 (16 ounces) can chili beans, drained

3 cups tortilla chips, crushed

2 cups sour cream

1 (2 ounces) can slice black olives, drained

1/2 cup chopped green onion

1/2 cup chopped fresh tomato

2 cups shredded Cheddar cheese

Kitchen Equipment:

oven

9x13 baking dish

Directions:

Prepare oven to 350 degrees Fahrenheit (175 degrees Celsius).

In a large fish over medium heat, cook the meat so that it is no longer pink. Add the sauce, reduce the heat and simmer for 20 minutes or until the liquid is absorbed. Add beans and heat.

Sprinkle a 9x13 baking dish with oil spray. Pour the chopped tortillas into the pan and then place the meat mixture on it. Pour sour cream over meat and sprinkle with olives, green onions, and tomatoes. Top with cheddar cheese.

Bake in preheated oven for 30 minutes or until hot and bubbly.

Nutrition:

Fat 43.7 - **Carbohydrates** 32.8 - **Protein** 31.7g

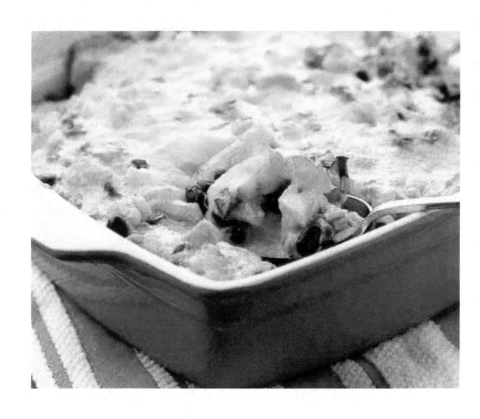

48. MICROWAVED FISH AND ASPARAGUS WITH TARRAGON MUSTARD SAUCE

Preparation Time: 10 minutes

Cooking Time: 20 minutes

Servings: 2

Ingredients

12 ounces (340 g) fish fillets—whiting, tilapia, sole, flounder, or any kind of white fish

10 asparagus spears

2 tablespoons (30 g) sour cream

1 tablespoon (15 g) mayonnaise

¼ teaspoon dried tarragon

½ teaspoon Dijon or spicy brown mustard

Kitchen Equipment:

large plate

microwave

pie plate

Directions:

Draw the bottom of the asparagus spears and cut them naturally. Put the asparagus on a large glass plate, add 1 teaspoon (15 ml) of water and cover with a plate. Microwave for 3 minutes.

While the asparagus is in the microwave, mix sour, mayonnaise, tarragon and mustard together.

Remove the asparagus from the microwave oven, remove it from the pie plate and set aside. Drain the water from the runway. Put the fish fillet in it

Peel the pie plate and spread 2 tablespoons (30 ml) cream mixture on them and cover the pie again and place the fish in the microwave for 3 to 4 minutes. Open the oven, remove the plate from the top of the pie plate and place the asparagus on top of the fish. Cover the pie plate again and cook for another 1-2 minutes.

Remove the pie plate from the microwave oven and remove the plate. Put the fish and asparagus on a serving platter. Chop any boiled sauce on a plate over fish and asparagus. Melt each with reserved sauce and serve.

Nutrition:

Carbs 4g - **Protein** 33g - **Fat** 17g

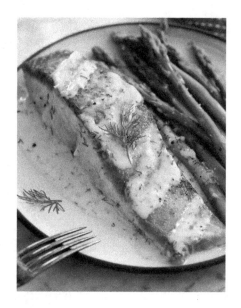

49. Hearty Hot Cereal with Berries

Preparation Time: 10 minutes

Cooking Time: 5 minutes

Servings: 4

Ingredients

4 cups of water

2 tablespoons honey

½ teaspoon salt

½ cup fresh blueberries

2 cups whole rolled oats

½ cup fresh raspberries

½ cup chopped walnuts

cup low-fat milk

teaspoons flaxseed

Kitchen Equipment:

Medium saucepan

Directions:

Boil water over high heat and stir in the salt in a medium saucepan. Stir in the oats, walnuts, and flaxseed, then reduce the heat to low and cover — Cook for 16 to 20 minutes, or until the oatmeal reaches the desired consistency.

Divide the oatmeal between 4 deep bowls and top each with 2 tablespoons of both blueberries and raspberries. Add ½ cup milk to each bowl and serve.

Nutrition: - **Fat** 15g - **Carbohydrates** 17g - **Protein** 19g

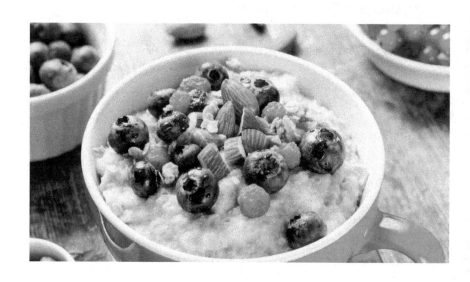

50. Protein Power Sweet Potatoes

Preparation Time: 15 minutes

Cooking Time: 10 minutes

Servings: 2

Ingredients

2 medium sweet potatoes

6 ounces plain Greek yogurt

½ teaspoon salt

1/3 cup dried cranberries

¼ teaspoon freshly ground black pepper

Kitchen Equipment:

oven

cooking plate

medium bowl

Directions:

Prepare the oven at 400 degrees F and prick the sweet potatoes several times. Place them on a cooking plate and cook for 40 to 45 minutes, or until you can easily pierce them with a fork.

Cut the potatoes in half and wrap the meat in a medium bowl and keep the skin healthy.

Add the salt, pepper, yogurt, and cranberries to the bowl and mix well with a fork.

Return the mixture back into the potato skins and serve warm.

Nutrition:

Fat 11g - **Carbohydrates** 15g - **Protein** 18g

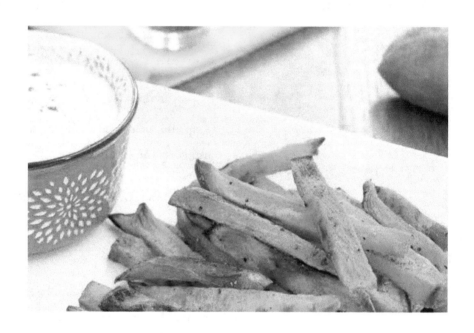

CPSIA information can be obtained
at www.ICGtesting.com
Printed in the USA
BVHW091423070621
608934BV00003B/1181